HIGHER ROAD PUBLISHING LLC

Brush, Floss, Thrive: Your Basic Guide to a Healthy Smile and Vibrant Well-Being

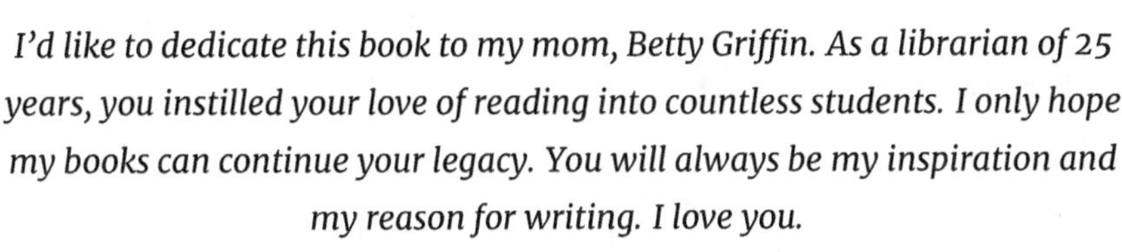

I'd like to dedicate this book to my mom, Betty Griffin. As a librarian of 25 years, you instilled your love of reading into countless students. I only hope my books can continue your legacy. You will always be my inspiration and my reason for writing. I love you.

To my oldest, Damian, may you always pursue your passions and follow your dreams. Thank you for encouraging me to find my own. To my Mason, may you never lose the joy and sparkle in your eyes. I love you both more than life.

Contents

1

Introduction

How many of you have heard that flossing increases your life expectancy? How many of you dismiss this statement as a myth? What if I told you..it's true?

As a Registered Dental Hygienist of 12+ years, I have discovered that there is an essential need for widespread basic education relating to oral health, and an even greater need for people to understand that their oral health is not just connected to overall health, but directly correlated. I will explain why, in my opinion, taking care of your mouth is the FIRST defense in helping to maintain your health and extend your life.

This book is intended to be the ultimate easy-to-read guide to help every single person with a mouth to understand the very important basics of taking care of your body through oral hygiene, dental care and overall healthy living. It includes pictures of common issues and explains what, why and how we do what we do at the dentist office and how to combat the common anxiety caused by the thoughts of what may happen at your dental appointments. I will explain common procedures and how maintaining your oral health at home is just as important to your health as exercising and eating healthy, and how regular visits to your dentist (and especially your dental hygienist) is just as important as seeing your medical doctor. I will be using this book as a supplemental tool in my practice to show patients that the dental world doesn't have to be scary or overwhelming, and I hope you come to the same conclusion.

As a dental professional, my favorite part of my job is connecting with my patients. I hope you can trust me to provide enlightening information that will empower you to take control of your health, starting with your smile. Everyone deserves to feel confident, and when someone has a healthy and happy smile, they can light up the world.

So let's get started and Brush, Floss and THRIVE!

What Dental Professionals Want our Patients to Know

So, you're thinking about making a dental appointment? Good, do it! But then what? Does your anxiety rise just thinking about the day you have to actually show up? Have you had a negative experience with a dentist in the past? The sad truth is, so many people have. Dentistry has not always been what it is today, and white-coat syndrome is real. The biggest hurdle for most people, in my opinion, is overcoming the anxiety that rises in us when we worry that what we will experience will be scary or painful. But, if you consider the fact that heart disease, stroke, diabetes and dementia are among the top ten deadliest diseases in the world, then neglecting our oral health seems much scarier when you become aware of the correlation between them. We know taking care of ourselves is vitally important to prevent or manage these diseases. Therefore, I urge you to decide that your fear is not worth sacrificing your health. Take the leap and make the appointment.

I promise that the vast majority of dentists and dental professionals want to help you. This is your reminder, that YOU are your own advocate when it comes to your health and your family's health. If you find yourself at a dental office, where you are uncomfortable or feel that your very best interests are not being considered or taken seriously, speak up or find one that is right for you. Do not hesitate to do what is best for you! That is what this book is about, right?

When the day comes, and you pull up to the office for your appointment, I encourage you to have a positive mindset. Most dental offices have one or more dentists, hygienists, assistants, front desk staff, and an office manager. These all have different duties and skill sets. Each of them has chosen to work in the public service industry, meaning we care about your health, safety and well-being. We all have bad days, of course, but for the most part I truly believe that my fellow professionals feel the same way I do, and want to help you.

Which brings me to what to expect at an initial appointment with your dentist. You pull up with a positive mindset and walk up to the front desk to get checked in. The first thing the front desk wants you to know is, we hate insurance too! Ask anyone in the medical field, insurance is not commonly anyone's friend. If you have insurance, the best tip I can give is to call your insurance prior to your appointment and find out exactly what they cover at your dentist. With or without insurance, the front desk and your whole dental team wants you to know that we understand that finances and paying for services is sometimes another cause for anxiety and stress. We understand that living in today's world is more expensive than it has ever been, and prioritizing your teeth is not always easy. Please respect your office's payment policies, but have hope that there are options. Recently, many medical and dental offices are offering financing through outside sources and this can be very helpful to many people that live on a budget, so don't hesitate to ask the front desk about your options.

At some point, before anything else, a medical history is performed to check for contraindications to dental treatment. I will review these contraindications in more detail in a later chapter, but we ask you to be very honest and thorough on your medical history. Sometimes vital signs are checked to verify the current state of health of a patient.

Commonly, the first step in a treatment plan for any new patient includes radiographs, also known as x-rays, of the mouth and teeth. These x-rays, along with a visual exam, help the dentist diagnose any abnormalities of the mouth or teeth during an exam. These abnormalities include, but are not limited to, bone loss around the teeth, decay (also known as dental caries or cavities) of the teeth, and infections of the teeth and surrounding structures.

A dental prophylaxis, or a cleaning is recommended as one of the first treatments to complete at the dentist. For many people, your dental hygienist is who you may spend most of your time with at the dentist office. We are certified, registered and extensively trained to give you the best tools, tips and tricks to maintain a healthy smile. We are dedicated to helping our patients learn and understand how important it is to prioritize their oral health. Coming only second to the regular home care of your teeth, we are your first line of defense against oral disease. We will ask you what issues you have had with your teeth and work to understand your dental history and address any current issues. We perform oral cancer screenings, periodontal charting to check for diseases of the gums (such as gingivitis or periodontitis), dental cleanings (or prophys, short for prophylaxis), and scaling and root planing procedures (commonly shortened to SRPs). It is highly recommended that you see your dental hygienist every six months for a regular cleaning and to get x-rays once a year. This will help you maintain your oral health by preventing or managing any gum disease and bring attention to any areas of concern. We may also remind you to try to have good habits at home, including brushing at least twice a day for a full two minutes and flossing once a day, before bed. There are also many different products to help people clean difficult to reach areas or do a more thorough job cleaning your teeth at home, so feel free to ask your hygienist for tips and tricks for your specific needs. For example, an electric toothbrush is always a good idea.

Typically after your dental cleaning is complete, the dentist will be called in to do a full mouth exam. During the exam, the dentist will check the teeth for cavities, or decay of the teeth. He will check the soft tissues, such as your cheeks, tongue and palate, for any signs of abnormalities and ask you what your chief concerns are. Together with your dentist and dental team, we will make a treatment plan for anything necessary to obtain, maintain, or sustain a healthy smile that you will be proud of for years to come.

Lastly, I will take this opportunity to say that as a dental professional, we all truly appreciate your patience. I know we have all had experiences with doctors' offices where we had to wait a while on someone or something. Dental is the same. We are here to help you, but we are human. Sometimes the day's schedule does not go as expected, and we all have bad days, but please treat your dental professionals as you would like to be treated. It helps us help you, and we truly want to establish and maintain good relationships with our patients so we can do everything we can to do our part in helping you thrive, starting with your oral health. So let's get started!

3

Gingivitis vs. Periodontal Disease

Gingivitis and periodontitis, or periodontal disease, are inflammatory diseases of the gums. The most common cause of these diseases is poor oral hygiene. When we eat and drink, debris gets trapped in between the teeth and in the space between the teeth and the gums surrounding the teeth. This space is called the sulcus. When debris is not removed by regular brushing and flossing, it causes bacteria to grow and plaque and calculus (or tartar) to form on the teeth. This bacteria releases toxins that attack the teeth and gums. This is why it is very important to try to prevent these diseases before they start.

The difference between the two types is the severity and progression of the gum disease. Healthy gums are firm and fit tightly around the teeth. They usually don't bleed during brushing and are normally a light pink color, but can range from dark pink to brown in some people. Gingivitis is very common and is characterized by swelling or puffiness of the gums, and especially bleeding upon brushing or flossing. This is reversible and with regular visits to your dental hygienist and good home care, the gingiva can normally be returned to a healthy state.

Periodontitis is a more severe form of gum disease. This involves swollen and bleeding gums as well, but also shows evidence of recession and bone loss. Recession is when the gums are irritated or damaged from the bacterial toxins in plaque and tartar to the point where they start pulling up and away from the teeth, exposing the root section of the tooth. This means that the bone and gums that support your teeth are deteriorating and disappearing. This is irreversible and could eventually cause the teeth to become loose and infections are more likely.

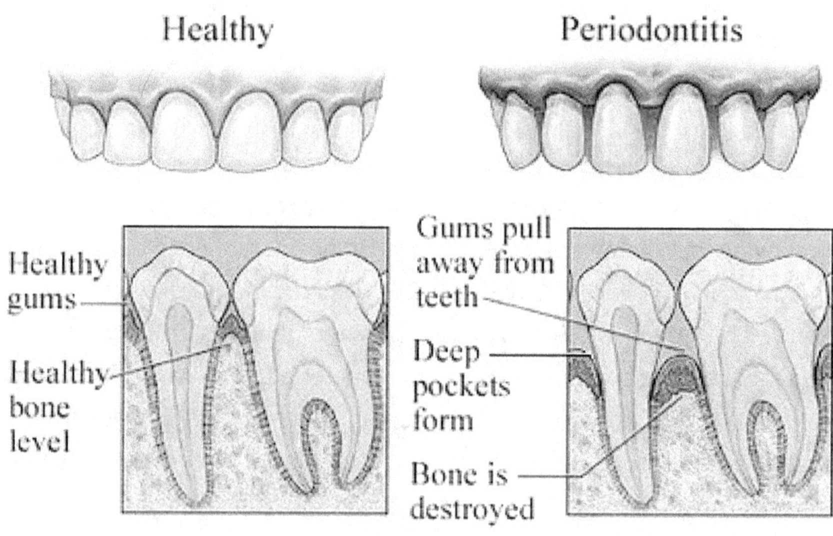

Diagram of Healthy vs. Diseased Gingiva

To diagnose these diseases a dental hygienist completes a periodontal chart with an instrument called a dental probe. This involves measuring the sulcus, or the space between the gums and the teeth. Between 1-3mm is considered healthy, or within normal limits. Anything above 4 is considered gum disease, but whether it is gingivitis or periodontitis is determined by the amount of recession and bone loss involved.

Thankfully, there is a treatment for periodontal disease that is recommended for patients called a scaling and root planing procedure. The procedure, also known as a deep cleaning, helps ensure that we give the patient their best chance at getting back to a healthy gingival state. For this type of cleaning, we anesthetize one quadrant, or a quarter section, of the mouth at a time and focus solely on removing plaque and calculus from the teeth in that section where it has gathered under the gums and around the teeth. We smooth the root surfaces and clear the debris, so that the gums can have their best chance at healing and getting back to a manageable and healthy state. The goal of this treatment is to stop or slow the disease progression to prevent tooth loss for as long as possible. Once treatment is completed in all four quadrants, it is recommended that you return every three months for a periodontal maintenance appointment. A hygienist will update your periodontal chart with new measurements that will hopefully indicate that your gums are healing. Periodontal disease is irreversible, but with this type of treatment, followed by good home care and regular follow up visits, the disease can be stabilized with the goal of extending the life of the teeth for years to come.

4

Other Dental Treatments

Besides regular cleanings and exams, there are many other common dental treatments to help maintain the health of your teeth. During a dental exam, a dentist will go tooth by tooth, which are numbered one through thirty-two, and make a chart of what treatment you may need. In this chapter we'll cover what common dental issues require which types of treatment.

First, your teeth have their very own anatomy. A very strong outer layer, called enamel, forms the covering that protects our teeth. If this enamel is compromised by decay or a break (or fracture) of the tooth and the inner layer of the tooth, called dentin, is exposed, this warrants the need for a filling. If the decay enters the innermost layer of the tooth, which is the pulp chamber, the blood vessels and nerves are likely to develop infection. This will require a root canal treatment.

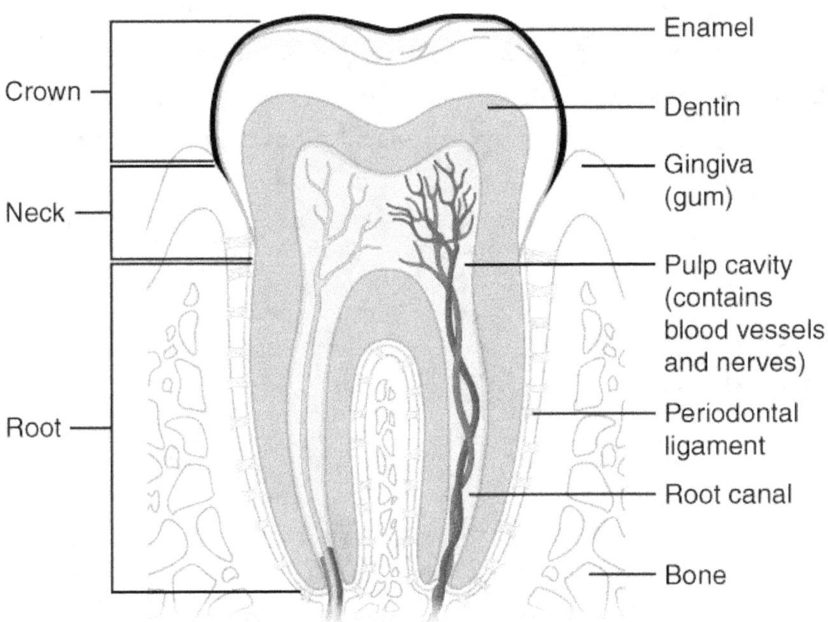

Diagram of Tooth Anatomy

The most common dental problem that almost everyone faces at some point in their lives is tooth decay. Cavities are caused when bacteria in your mouth produce acids that dissolve the tooth enamel over time. When a dentist removes the decayed portion of the tooth, fillings are used to replace the lost tooth structure. The size of a filling depends on the size of the cavity. Teeth have different surfaces, which help us signify what part of the tooth needs a filling. These are the mesial, distal, buccal/facial, lingual and occlusal surfaces. During a filling procedure, the tooth area on which the decay is present is anesthetized, or numbed, and the dentist will use different sized burs to remove the decayed tooth surface. Tooth colored composite filling material is placed where tooth structure used to be and hardened with a curing light. In the past, silver colored fillings, called amalgams, were commonly used for fillings, but today's filling material is very strong and more aesthetically pleasing. Usually the need for a filling is indicated by sensitivity to hot or cold, brushing or touching the area, and visual abnormalities or dark places on the teeth.

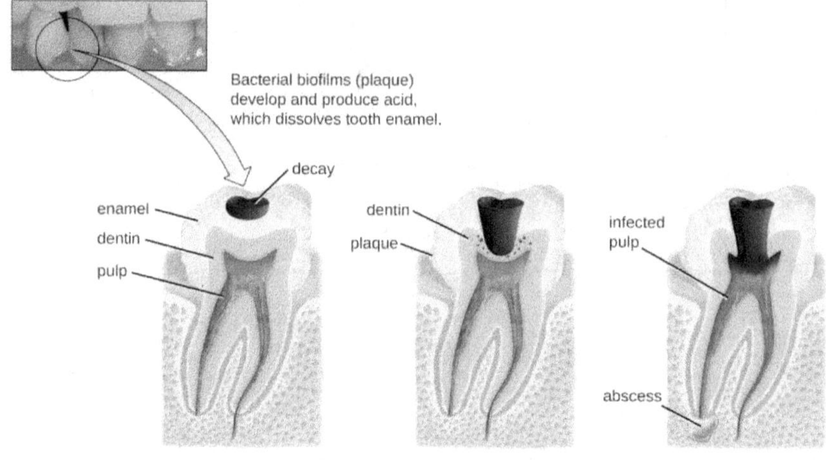

Diagram of a Filling

If a tooth is decayed or even broken to the point that a dentist feels that the remaining tooth structure would not be able to retain a filling, a crown may be recommended. A crown, or cap, is placed over a tooth that does not have much tooth structure left and would be at risk of breaking if treated by a filling. It covers, or caps, the remaining tooth structure to stabilize that tooth. The crowns of today are normally made of a strong porcelain material that resembles a real tooth, but many people still have silver crowns, and some even gold.

A more serious and usually more urgent issue commonly seen at the dentist is a toothache, or abscess. These abscesses are infections caused when bacteria enters the pulp of the tooth and are usually reported as very painful to pressure, or on its own. This usually causes swelling of the jaw or affected area. Because this problem indicates infection around the root tip of the afflicted tooth, it is normally treated by first prescribing the patient antibiotics. After the antibiotic regimen has been completed, the patient has the option of removing the tooth by extraction, or a root canal treatment. A root canal treatment is when the pulp inside the root canals of the teeth is removed and replaced with a medicated filling material. The tooth is resealed and usually crowned later on to stabilize the tooth after a root canal. There is no guarantee that a tooth with a root canal will not get re-infected later on, but this is usually a successful treatment for an abscessed tooth that the patient desires to save. Sometimes, the patient may decide to opt out of a root canal, simply due to cost or fear of reinfection.

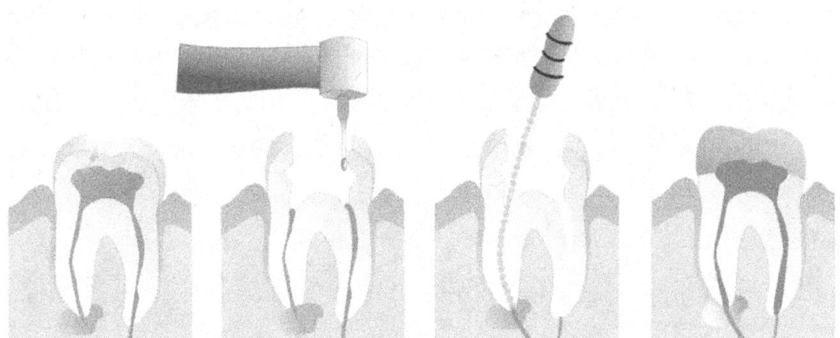

Diagram of Root Canal Treatment

An extraction is an option for a tooth that has been infected, or is broken or decayed to the point that it does not have enough tooth structure remaining to save it. These can be simple extractions, or if sutures of the gums are involved due to a difficult removal of a tooth, it is called a surgical extraction. Many times, third molars, or wisdom teeth require surgical extractions due to the position of the teeth and how they are commonly impacted under gum tissue and bone.

Once a tooth has been removed, there are usually options to replace the tooth in the space it once was. One option is a bridge. A bridge is an appliance that utilizes placing a crown on the teeth on both sides of the missing tooth. These crowns are attached to a false tooth in the middle, creating essentially a bridge that covers that space. It is cemented in place and is meant to be a permanent solution to replacing missing teeth. A drawback to a bridge is that it affects the teeth on either side of the space, and may cause problems in the future for those teeth if not maintained and kept clean. Another permanent option is a dental implant. An implant is an artificial tooth root that is screwed into the bone where a tooth was removed. A crown, bridge or even partials and dentures can be attached to an implant. A drawback to an implant is that you have to wait up to six months after an extraction to have it placed. This is due to the time it takes for the bone where the tooth was removed to regrow to a state that it can support an implant.

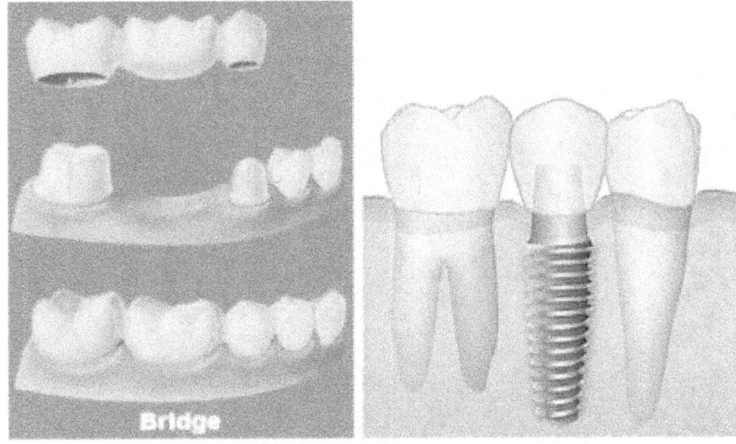

Diagram of Bridge vs. Implant

Lastly, there are different types of removable appliances to replace multiple missing teeth. Partials are recommended as an option for people missing multiple teeth and are made of either an acrylic resin material or a combination of this resin material and metal. Resin partials are usually more natural looking, but partials with metal clasps usually last longer and may fit better.

These are the most common procedures performed at most dental offices. Thankfully, there are many options for most dental ailments, so if a tooth is hurting, do not hesitate to see your dentist. It is not healthy for infection to stay in the body and no one should have to withstand the pain of a toothache for longer than necessary.

5

Specialty Dentistry

Beyond general dentistry there is a wide range of dentists that specialize in certain treatment areas. This chapter will go over the different types of specialty dentists and what they do.

A pedodontist is a dentist that specializes in treating babies, children, or young people. They do many of the same treatments as a general dentist, but often have different techniques to help young children manage any fears they may have going into dental procedures. Pedodontists often see sick, disabled or special needs children and can also use general anesthesia for children in need of extensive dental work, or those that are too afraid to be awake during a procedure.

Orthodontists are dentists that usually do not perform regular dental procedures, but focus more on the treatments used to straighten the teeth and fix the alignment of the jaw. Most patients that have orthodontic treatment are children, due to the fact that when people are younger, their jaws and teeth are easier to move if malaligned from development, but some adults seek treatment stating that their parents or caregivers were not able or interested in straightening their teeth. For many years, the traditional methods of orthodontics included metal brackets and wires. Over time, the methods have gone to clear brackets and even clear retainer systems, such as Invisalign, to help with the aesthetic factor of having braces. There are many benefits to having straight teeth and an aligned jaw that comes together in what is called normal occlusion when biting normally on our back teeth. The obvious one, is the aesthetic benefit, meaning how it looks nice when someone has straight teeth, but the less obvious benefits include prevention of TMJ disease. TMJ is the temporomandibular joint that enables us to open and close our mouths. If this joint deteriorates over time it can be very painful for the patient, and sometimes causes popping and locking of the jaw. This is caused when the teeth are not coming together properly and therefore puts undue pressure on the joint. If the teeth are straightened to normal occlusion at a young age it can help prevent this painful disease. It can also prevent the teeth from wearing on each other unnecessarily and causing wear of the chewing surfaces over time. Straighter teeth are also normally much easier for the patient to brush and floss, therefore preventing tooth decay. The drawbacks of orthodontic treatment include the price of treatment and the fact that the patient has to be able to follow strict oral hygiene instructions to prevent problems, like decay around the orthodontic brackets and appliances.

Periodontists are dentists specializing in periodontal disease, like the gum diseases discussed earlier. They not only usually have hygienists that can complete scaling and root planing procedures, but they specialize in tissue grafting and bone grafting procedures. These extensive procedures involve using the patient's own tissue from a donor site on their palate, and placing the tissue over areas of recession, or a cadaver bone to replace lost bone structure. This can give patients a chance at replacing lost gingival tissue and bone support around teeth to extend the life of those teeth. Periodontists also specialize in placing implants and work in conjunction with the patient's general dentist to maintain the best outcomes for someone with periodontal issues.

An endodontist is a dentist that specializes in root canal treatments. Once a tooth becomes infected, treatment of the affected tooth pulp is required and endodontists perform these procedures every day. Many general dentists perform root canal treatments, but may refer a patient to an endodontist if a certain tooth has pulp canals that may be difficult to access and treat.

An oral and maxillofacial surgeon is a dentist that specializes in oral surgeries, such as surgical or difficult extractions. They are able to place patients under general anesthesia and remove multiple teeth at once. Patients are often referred to oral surgeons by general dentists for the removal of all the wisdom teeth, or third molars, at once. Oral and maxillofacial surgeons can also specialize in areas such as radiology and pathology, if a patient has an area of concern beyond the scope of a general dentist.

In summary, your general dentist can treat many dental problems but specialty dentists have many years of training in their field and are highly equipped to handle any complicated or complex problem that may arise.

6

Contraindications to Dental Treatment

There are only a few reasons why a dentist may tell you it is not a good time for you as a patient to receive dental treatment. I'll discuss these contraindications for treatment and why they exist. This is the main reason that a medical history assessment is required when you visit a dentist. This assessment should ideally include your current medical conditions and any plans for treatment. If there is a history of any chronic conditions, such as diabetes, are those conditions being managed? A list of current medications is needed as well. We as dental professionals want to make sure we provide the safest and best care to you as an individual.

People often wonder if pregnancy is a reason to postpone dental work, or if it is safe to see your dentist or hygienist while pregnant. The answer is yes. In fact, it is actually very important for a woman to maintain her oral health during pregnancy because studies have linked gum disease to preterm birth and low birth weight. It is also important to prevent any infections that could possibly cross the placenta and affect the baby. Pregnant women should maintain good home care and keep their regular dental cleaning appointments to help prevent gum disease, which is common due to hormonal changes. If morning sickness is often a problem during pregnancy, erosion of the tooth enamel from the stomach acid in vomit becomes a concern. To prevent erosion of your teeth if you experience morning sickness, it is recommended that you rinse with baking soda mixed with water and then wait thirty minutes or so to brush. If any dental work is needed during pregnancy, it is recommended that it be performed during the second trimester, or to wait until after delivery if possible and safe to do so, though it is often safe to do so at other times during pregnancy as well. Your dentist and OB/GYN will work with you to decide what is ideal for your needs.

Another contraindication to dental treatment would be a recent heart attack, meaning within the last six weeks. If the patient has had a stent placed, an organ transplant, or other heart surgery, elective dental treatment should wait six months. It is also wise to complete any dental treatment necessary before a patient starts undergoing head and neck radiation therapy, to help prevent problems during their treatment. On the other hand, a patient can receive routine dental treatment during chemotherapy, provided their oncologist gives their approval, or clearance, to do so.

It used to be a very common practice to give patients with certain medical conditions antibiotics prior to any dental treatment to prevent any infections. These were patients with prosthetic joint implants or heart disease that puts them at risk for infective endocarditis. More recently, it has been determined that the risk of adverse reactions to antibiotics and development of antibiotic-resistant bacteria has been shown to be greater than the benefit to the patient. Therefore, prophylactic antibiotics are no longer recommended unless there are special circumstances such as a history of infection or if the patient is immunocompromised.

Lastly, a class of antiresorptive medicine used for treatment of osteoporosis in women called bisphosphonates may hinder the regrowth of bone if a patient has a tooth extracted. Some medications, such as beta blockers, may interact with the dental anesthetic, while others may cause dry mouth, so it is helpful to give your dentist a thorough medical history and list of medications.

When in doubt about whether it is okay to see your dentist while other health issues are present, it is always a good idea to get clearance before starting dental treatment from your medical doctor or specialist. When your medical and dental teams communicate and work together, your total body health is considered and can be maintained and hopefully even improved.

7

Relation Between Nutrition and Oral Health

Most of us understand that eating candy all the time and never brushing our teeth would cause cavities. But I'll explain how our nutrition affects our oral health in more ways than you might expect. I'll talk about what vitamins and minerals our teeth need and the things that are harmful.

First and foremost, fluoride is a mineral that has long been shown to help in the fight against cavities, but you may be surprised to learn that it was first discovered to be helpful through the discovery that too much of it was actually harmful. Fluoride was originally discovered through the investigation of brown staining on children's teeth. It was eventually determined that high levels of fluoride in the drinking water in some areas of the United States was the cause. In 1901, a young dentist named Dr. Frederick McKay was researching why brown stains were appearing on young children's teeth in Colorado and other areas across the states. Interestingly, Dr. McKay also noticed that these stained teeth were highly resistant to tooth decay. In 1931, it was finally discovered through a new water testing analysis method that fluoride was the cause of the brown staining, now known as fluorosis. By the late 1930s, a way to measure fluoride levels in drinking water was discovered and a safe level was determined. 1.0 parts per million, or 1.0ppm, of fluoride in drinking water was considered to be a safe level that would not cause fluorosis in the developing teeth of children, but would indeed aid in the prevention of dental cavities. In 1945, after much consideration, the city of Grand Rapids, Michigan led the way and was the first city to fluoridate its public water supply. The effects revolutionized the world of dentistry. The prevalence of tooth decay dropped by 60% in children born after fluoride was added to the water supply. Now the focus in dentistry could shift from maintaining or removing problem teeth, to hopefully preventing the decay of those teeth in the first place. Today, water fluoridation has become common and now benefits most Americans. Fluoride is also used in most toothpastes and many schools still implement fluoride rinse programs for their students. As a dental professional, I am thankful that the benefits of fluoride for our teeth were discovered and that tooth decay is now considered a preventable disease.

Along with fluoride, other vitamins and minerals are vital to the healthy development of our teeth. It is important, especially in children with developing permanent teeth to get a nutritious diet full of these vitamins and minerals. A multivitamin is a good supplement to our diet, whether we're children or adults because most of us do not get the daily recommended amount of these vitamins and minerals. The main minerals that are good for our teeth are calcium and phosphorus. These, along with Vitamin A, help protect and rebuild tooth enamel. Vitamin C aids in keeping our gums healthy and healing. You can find many sources of these vitamins and minerals. Calcium is found in milk, cheese, yogurt and almonds just to name a few and look for protein-rich foods, such as meat, fish and eggs to get more phosphorus. Fruits and vegetables are great for our teeth and our bodies, due to them being high in vitamins and fiber. A well rounded diet full of nutrient rich foods and low in added sugars will benefit your teeth and overall health for your whole life, especially if these habits are started early in life.

Now, we know that the opposite is just as true. Any food or drinks that are high in sugar or have higher acidity levels can cause tooth decay if not consumed in moderation. Bacteria in the plaque formed by what we eat and drink, uses this sugar and acid to attack and deteriorate the tooth enamel, causing cavities. This includes soda or other sweetened beverages and foods like cakes and candies. This is especially true if we snack or sip on sugary foods or drinks throughout the day. Fluoridated water is the best thing you can have in between meals, saving the food and other drinks for mealtime only. If we neglect our bodies by not paying attention to what we put in them, it can have devastating effects on our oral health and our overall health. Processed foods high in salts and sugars have almost no nutritional benefits and often cause issues with our health far beyond our teeth.

Along with eating healthy and being conscious of what we drink, there are many harmful effects associated with tobacco and alcohol consumption. Oral cancer is very serious and has been proven to be linked to tobacco usage. Smoking cigarettes and chewing smokeless tobacco not only causes bad breath and the discoloration of teeth, but can cause the breakdown of gum tissues and bone support for your teeth. This often results in cavities, periodontal disease and tooth loss in the future. It is highly discouraged to use these products and there are many smoking cessation resources if you are interested in quitting. Vaping is relatively new compared to tobacco products, but negative effects on your oral health are also a concern. Lastly, alcohol can cause dry mouth, is usually acidic and may be high in sugar so it is recommended to limit your intake. Lacking healthy nutrition and consuming tobacco and alcohol are leading contributing factors for inflammation and infection in the body. Taking care of your oral health by getting the proper nutrition will only have positive effects on your overall health and well-being.

8

Diabetes and Oral Health

It has been proven through many studies over time that the health of our mouths is directly related to our overall health. Diabetes, heart disease, obesity, and Alzheimer's disease are just a few that have been linked to oral health. I will briefly explain how one affects the other and what we need to do to combat these diseases through regular dental care.

Diabetes is one of the main diseases that has been linked to oral disease. It is a metabolic disorder that is caused when the body does not produce enough insulin or is insulin-resistant. This causes high blood sugar for long periods of time and when not managed well can also cause severe complications, such as nerve damage, eye problems, high blood pressure and even heart problems or strokes. Your oral health is at risk when you have diabetes type one, two or even gestational diabetes (which develops during pregnancy) because this disease reduces the body's ability to resist and fight infection. Therefore, gum disease is commonly seen in patients with diabetes and often is more severe. But thankfully, it has been shown that with regular periodontal care, such as regular cleanings or the scaling and root planing procedures discussed earlier, diabetes can be better managed and controlled. Research has shown that blood sugar levels are harder to control in people with gum disease, so it becomes a negative cycle of disease when left unmanaged. It is vital for someone with diabetes to see their dental hygienist on a regular basis to record any changes to your gums or catch any development of gum disease early, and help manage periodontal disease if already present.

Together with blood sugar management through proper diet and medication, regular dental visits and daily home care of your teeth with regular brushing and flossing will be the main defense against developing oral problems as a result of diabetes. With a healthy mouth, and awareness of the connection between them, diabetes can be more easily managed to help you achieve a full, healthy life.

9

Heart Disease and Oral Health

Another disease that has been closely linked with our oral health is cardiovascular disease, or heart disease. Heart disease is a broad term for conditions of the heart that affect how it functions and how the blood flows through it. It is known that certain kinds of bacteria cause certain oral problems. For example, cavities are mainly caused by streptococcus mutans bacteria, gingivitis is usually caused by streptococcus and actinomyces bacteria and periodontal disease is caused by these strains, along with the addition of porphyromonas bacteria species. Heart disease is thought to be connected to these oral diseases because it has been shown that the same bacteria that causes infection and inflammation in the mouth also lead to the clogged arteries that cause the heart attacks and strokes associated with heart disease.

Infective endocarditis is a life-threatening heart condition that has been connected to oral disease. Endocarditis is a condition in which the inner lining of your endocardium, or heart chambers or valves, develops an infection This is typically caused when bacteria from other areas of the body travel through your bloodstream into your heart. This includes bacteria from your mouth, and when left untreated endocarditis can cause major damage or completely destroy the heart valves. Therefore, the more you can control the bacteria in your mouth, the less that bacteria has a chance to spread and affect other areas of your body.

Symptoms of heart problems include aching muscles, chest pains, fatigue, shortness of breath, swelling or irregular heart sounds. If you experience any of these symptoms please seek medical attention right away.

10

Other Chronic Diseases and Oral Health

Along with diabetes and heart disease, many other diseases have been proven to have a connection to the health of our mouths. The biggest link between chronic disease and oral health is inflammation. As discussed earlier, nutrition is very important to our bodies and our oral health. Without proper nutrition, our bodies are less able to fight this inflammation and the likelihood of infection or disease is higher. Therefore, eating disorders and obesity along with periodontal disease are known risk factors contributing to chronic inflammation and the diseases associated with it. This proves that eating healthy and having good oral health habits, can have a positive impact on the longevity and quality of your life.

Anxiety and depression are often overlooked conditions that can have an affect on our mouths. It is understandable that everyone becomes stressed sometimes, and that anxiety and depression can have negative effects on our self-care habits, including brushing and flossing. But beyond these behavioral changes, stress also causes our cortisol levels to increase. When the level of this naturally occurring hormone rises in our bodies, it causes the weakening of our immune systems, which can lead to inflammation and infection. Noticing a pattern here? Stress along with medications used to treat anxiety and depression can also cause dry mouth, which then contributes to plaque formation and development of cavities, so it is important to be aware of these side effects and to strive to have good oral hygiene at home and visit your dentist regularly, even when you may not be feeling your best.

Osteoporosis is a disease that causes bones to become weak and brittle and often results in serious bone fractures of the hips or spine. The effects of osteoporosis become a problem for our oral health if we need a tooth extracted or would like an implant placed, due to the antiresorptive medications used to treat this disease. These medications have been associated with a condition known as osteonecrosis of the jaw, or ONJ. This rare but serious condition can occur without reason, but usually occurs after completion of surgical dental procedures and results in severe deterioration of the jawbone. It is vital that you tell your dentist all the medications you are taking so they can make an appropriate and safe treatment plan for your individual needs.

Dementia and Alzheimer's disease have been linked to poor oral health. Tooth loss for any reason has been shown to increase the likelihood of these diseases, and over time as these diseases progress a decline of oral health is usually observed in these patients affected by memory loss. If you are a caregiver of someone with dementia or Alzheimer's, it is highly recommended that you help these people with their oral care at home, as they may not be able to effectively remember to brush and floss.

Other diseases such as the herpes simplex virus and HIV/AIDS often cause painful ulcers in the mouth that may likely keep patients from performing proper home care, resulting in gum disease and tooth decay. These viruses cause the immune system to be compromised and can lower the body's ability to fight infection, making dental problems more likely to be severe. Warm salt water rinses for the mouth sores and antiviral medications are often prescribed to help manage the symptoms of these diseases.

Respiratory diseases, such as pneumonia, have been linked to the bacteria in our mouths. It is possible for certain bacteria to travel or be pulled into the respiratory tract and lungs and cause infection.

Kidney disease, rheumatoid arthritis and even certain cancers have also been linked to our oral health. So although it may seem that oral diseases should be isolated to the mouth, the relationship they have with the rest of the body has been repeatedly proven and should not be ignored. To manage chronic disease and inflammation and positively affect our general health, our oral health must be of top priority. Along with a healthy diet, and eliminating or limiting tobacco and alcohol use, having good oral health can greatly reduce the risk of many of these diseases. When you are aware of your health conditions and how they affect your oral health and vice versa, you have the power to change the future of your total body health by preventing or managing disease.

11

Holistic Approaches to Oral Health

Also known as alternative dentistry, holistic dentistry approaches and treats dental problems from the root cause by utilizing traditional methods along with whole body health, instead of only focusing on the symptoms of oral disease. Holistic dentistry is not a specialty, but is like traditional dentistry in that they both focus on the overall health of the mouth. Holistic dentistry, though, bases treatment on a set of core ideologies that take a more natural approach. These ideologies include removing outdated dental materials, such as old amalgam fillings which contain mercury, and replacing them with materials known to be healthier and more biocompatible with the body. This includes replacing fluoride with alternative methods of reducing the risk of cavities. They use nutrition as a key ingredient to prevent and even reverse dental disease. There is an emphasis on preventing and treating periodontal disease at the biological level and correcting malocclusion of the teeth. As a reminder, this is the teeth's position in the mouth, and when we optimize their ability to come together to function correctly and eliminate undue stress while chewing and talking, the risk of many future dental problems is greatly reduced.

Holistic dentists often collaborate with medical practitioners to improve the whole body health of the patient. They will often run specific diagnostic and biocompatibility tests to determine what treatments are the most safe and effective for the individual patient. They also take a thorough medical history, but usually ask for a detailed nutrition assessment as well and may give advice on where improvements can be made.

Traditional dental providers have often claimed that holistic dentistry is often not based on scientific fact, but if you agree with the core ideologies that holistic dentistry strives to uphold, to treat the whole body and the root causes of dental problems, then it may be for you. The Holistic Dental Association is a great resource for patients who would like to find dental providers who offer a more natural approach to dental care and treatment of disease.

12

Breaking Generational Cycles of Oral Neglect

For many years, dental health has not been a priority for previous generations and this neglect was passed down through the ages. Now that we are aware of the effects that oral disease can have on our bodies, and how chronic disease affects our dental health, teaching good oral habits to our young people should be considered nothing less than essential. From the time we are small children we are developing habits that we will keep for the rest of our lives. As parents, caregivers, teachers and authority figures, empowering our young people with knowledge about their mouths and bodies can lead them to take control of their health from an early age, with the hope that the risk for the chronic diseases we have discussed could be greatly reduced or even eliminated.

Children need help learning to effectively brush and floss their teeth. They generally need help with this up until the age of five or six, but this varies with the child's individual abilities. It is often recommended that a child as young as two to four years see a dentist, not only to check for any dental issues, but also to get them accustomed to coming to the dentist and relieve any future anxieties about visiting a dentist regularly. A pedodontist is a great option for children who may be fearful of the dentist or need more extensive dental work.

As an adult, the best thing we can do is set a good example for the children and young people around us. Displaying consideration for our own dental health and carrying out good oral care habits goes a long way in creating the desire in our children to follow in our footsteps. Be an example and make brushing and flossing a fun and regular habit, and hopefully that will continue for life. I hope this book reaches young people, through the adults in their lives that care about and want them to know how important their oral habits and health is to their well-being, for their entire lives. So pass it on to your children, family, friends, and everyone you know with a mouth. Oh, and please leave a review! Let's spread the word that one of the easiest and best ways to help us thrive in life is to take care of our oral health, so that future generations have their best chance at fighting these diseases.

13

Take Action

In summary, the following are some actions you can take that are highly recommended to support good oral health. Utilize the anti-cavity benefits of fluoride by drinking fluoridated water and brushing with a toothpaste containing fluoride. Strive to practice good oral hygiene every day by brushing thoroughly twice a day and flossing daily to prevent the buildup of plaque. Set a goal to visit your dentist at least once a year, but twice a year is recommended. Do not use tobacco products and seek help to quit if needed and limit alcoholic drinks. Put effort into eating healthy and managing health conditions to optimize oral health. Remember that many medications affect our oral health by causing dry mouth. If dry mouth is an issue for you, there are over-the-counter products that may be able to help that your dentist or doctor can recommend. Always drink plenty of water and chew sugar-free gum in between meals if possible. Lastly, remember to be a good example and if you are a caregiver or parent, help those who are not able to effectively brush and floss their teeth on their own.

14

Closing

As a dental professional turned author, I am happy to have the opportunity to reach people beyond the scope of my practice with what I hope will be a valuable resource for people to learn about and understand the basics of dentistry and dental care. Over many years, I have had conversations with countless people that simply have never been informed of the importance of regular dental visits, what a healthy mouth can do for the body and how to obtain and maintain a healthy smile. I hope to raise this awareness to the point where when people search on the internet, "how to extend your life expectancy" the list includes oral care at the very top.

Lastly, I have seen firsthand the devastating effects that neglecting their oral health can have on someone's self-image and self-esteem. Social anxiety is common to the point where people avoid socializing, or simply avoid smiling in social situations. This breaks my heart, but I have also seen how positive oral health can enhance an individual's mental and overall health. For this reason, I became a dental hygienist. To help people realize that they do not have to live in a cycle of bad health and suffering due to dental problems and to be a support in this journey of life that we all struggle with at times. It may seem odd, but regular visits to your dentist and dental hygienist is a vital part of your mental health and overall well-being. We as dental professionals are here to help you learn the best ways to take care of your unique mouth as an individual and show you that doing so, just might change your whole life.

I hope you feel enlightened and impassioned to begin a journey of health today that will have a positive impact on your health for the rest of your life, starting with your smile. Once again, I truly believe that everyone deserves to feel confident and happy in this life, and when someone has a healthy and happy smile, they can light up the world.

So I challenge you to love yourself and Brush, Floss and THRIVE!

15

Resources

Face Value Dental. (2019, January 16). How Oral Health Can Affect Overall Health. Retrieved August 27, 2023, from https://www.facevaluedental.com/how-oral-health-can-affect-overall-health#:~:text=Studies%20have%20also%20shown%20links%20between%20poor%20oral,linked%20to%20severe%20gum%20disease%20%28periodontitis%29%20More%20items

Pietrangelo, A. (2023, April 19). The Top 10 Deadliest Diseases (R. Ajmera MS, RD, Ed.). Healthline. Retrieved August 27, 2023, from https://www.healthline.com/health/top-10-deadliest-diseases

Mayo Clinic Staff. (2023, February 24). Periodontitis. Mayo Clinic. Retrieved August 27, 2023, from https://www.mayoclinic.org/diseases-conditions/periodontitis/symptoms-causes/syc-20354473

Professional, C. C. M. (2021, September 7). Root Canal:: What Is It, Diagnosis, Treatment, Side Effects and Recovery. Cleveland Clinic. Retrieved August 27, 2023, from https://my.clevelandclinic.org/health/treatments/21759-root-canal

Hill, A. (2023, August 2). Dental Specialties:: Compare Your Treatment
Options. NewMouth. Retrieved August 27, 2023, from https://www.new
mouth.com/dentistry/specialties/

American Pregnancy Association. (2021, December 9). Pregnancy and
Dental Work. Retrieved August 27, 2023, from https://americanpregna
ncy.org/healthy-pregnancy/is-it-safe/dental-work-and-pregnancy/

Herrick, K. R., MD, PhD, Terrio, J. M., DDS, & Herrick, C., DDS. (2021).
Medical Clearance for Common Dental Procedures. American Family
Physician, 104(5), 476–483. https://www.aafp.org/pubs/afp/issues/
2021/1100/p476.html

ADA. (2022, January 5). Antibiotic Prophylaxis Prior to Dental Cleanings.
American Dental Association. Retrieved August 27, 2023, from https://w
ww.ada.org/resources/research/science-and-research-institute/oral-
health-topics/antibiotic-prophylaxis

NIDCR. (2018, July). The Story of Fluoridation. National Institute of
Dental and Craniofacial Research. Retrieved August 27, 2023, from
https://www.nidcr.nih.gov/health-info/fluoride/the-story-of-fluorid
ation

Harvard T.H. Chan School of Public Health. (2022, December 2). Oral
health. The Nutrition Source. Retrieved August 27, 2023, from https://w
ww.hsph.harvard.edu/nutritionsource/oral-health/

Mayo Clinic Staff. (2021, October 28). Oral health: A Window to Your
Overall Health. Mayo Clinic. Retrieved August 27, 2023, from https://ww
w.mayoclinic.org/healthy-lifestyle/adult-health/in-depth/dental/art-
20047475

Bohn, J. A. G., BS, RDH, Haddlesey, C., BA, & McComas, M. J., [RDH, MS]. (2023, April 18). Holistic Dentistry: The Whole Approach to Oral Healthcare. Dimensions of Dental Hygiene | Magazine. Retrieved August 27, 2023, from https://dimensionsofdentalhygiene.com/article/holistic-dentistry-the-whole-approach-to-oral-healthcare/#:~:text=Holistic%20and%20traditional%20dentistry%20both%20address%20the%20health,treating%20periodontal%20diseases%20at%20their%20biological%20basis.%204

About the Author

Jami Yates is a Registered Dental Hygienist from southeast Missouri. She graduated with a Bachelor's in Health Science with an emphasis in Dental Hygiene and an Associate's Degree in Dental Hygiene from Missouri Southern State University in 2011. She has worked in the clinical setting for 12+ years and has always had a passion for helping people. She has two children, both boys ages 17 and 4 and loves spending quality time with her family and friends and traveling whenever possible.